I0096778

ISBN 978-1-998455-39-3 (Paperback)
ISBN 978-1-998455-40-9 (eBook)

Printed and bound in USA
Published by Loons Press

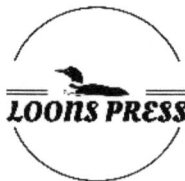

LOONS PRESS

A Holistic Approach

Table Of Contents

How To Manage Celiac Disease Naturally

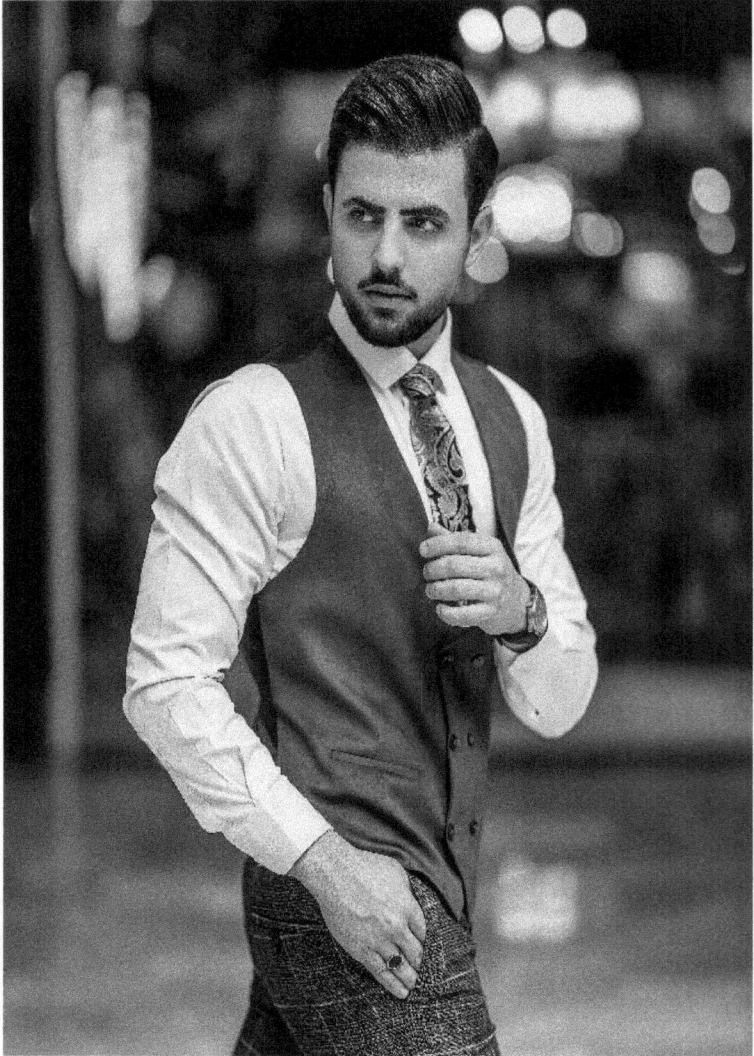

A Holistic Approach

Chapter 1

Understanding Celiac Disease

What is Celiac Disease?

Celiac disease is an autoimmune disorder that affects the small intestine. It is triggered by the ingestion of gluten, a protein found in wheat, barley, and rye. When someone with celiac disease consumes gluten, their immune system responds by attacking the lining of the small intestine. This can lead to a host of symptoms, including digestive issues, fatigue, skin problems, and nutrient deficiencies.

For people who have celiac disease, managing their condition naturally can be a game-changer. By following a gluten-free diet and incorporating holistic practices into their daily routine, individuals with celiac disease can experience significant improvements in their health and well-being. This approach focuses on healing the body from the inside out, addressing not just the symptoms of the disease but also the underlying causes.

One key aspect of managing celiac disease naturally is paying close attention to what goes into your body. This means avoiding gluten-containing foods like bread, pasta, and baked goods, as well as processed foods that may contain hidden sources of gluten. Instead, focus on whole, nutrient-dense foods like fruits, vegetables, lean proteins, and gluten-free grains. By nourishing your body with wholesome ingredients, you can support your gut health and reduce inflammation, which are crucial for managing celiac disease.

In addition to following a gluten-free diet, individuals with celiac disease can benefit from incorporating holistic practices such as stress management, mindfulness, and regular exercise into their daily routine.

Chronic stress can exacerbate symptoms of celiac disease, so finding ways to relax and unwind is essential for overall well-being. Mindfulness practices like meditation and deep breathing can help calm the nervous system and reduce inflammation in the body, while regular exercise can support immune function and improve digestion.

Overall, taking a holistic approach to managing celiac disease can lead to significant improvements in symptoms and quality of life. By focusing on nourishing your body with healthy foods, managing stress levels, and incorporating mindfulness practices and regular exercise into your routine, you can support your body's natural healing process and live well with celiac disease.

Remember, everyone's journey with celiac disease is unique, so it's important to listen to your body and work with a healthcare provider or holistic practitioner to develop a personalized plan that works for you.

Causes and Risk Factors

Celiac disease is an autoimmune disorder that affects the small intestine, causing a range of symptoms such as diarrhea, bloating, and fatigue. The main cause of celiac disease is the body's reaction to gluten, a protein found in wheat, barley, and rye. When someone with celiac disease consumes gluten, their immune system mistakenly attacks the lining of the small intestine, leading to inflammation and damage.

There are several risk factors that can increase the likelihood of developing celiac disease. Genetics play a significant role, as individuals with a family history of the condition are more likely to develop it themselves. Other risk factors include having other autoimmune disorders, such as Type 1 diabetes or thyroid disease, as well as certain genetic conditions like Down syndrome.

In addition to genetic factors, environmental triggers can also contribute to the development of celiac disease. For example, early exposure to gluten in infancy, certain infections, and stress have been linked to an increased risk of developing the condition. Additionally, factors such as a diet high in gluten-containing foods and a leaky gut can also increase the likelihood of celiac disease.

It's important to note that celiac disease can be triggered at any age, and symptoms can vary widely from person to person. Some individuals may experience severe symptoms, while others may have mild or even no symptoms at all. This variability makes it crucial for those with celiac disease to work closely with healthcare providers to manage their condition effectively.

While genetics and environmental factors play a role in the development of celiac disease, it's important to remember that the condition can be managed effectively through lifestyle changes and dietary modifications. By working with a healthcare provider and adopting a gluten-free diet, individuals with celiac disease can reduce inflammation, heal their gut, and improve their overall health and well-being. By understanding the causes and risk factors associated with celiac disease, those affected can take proactive steps to manage their condition naturally and live a healthy, fulfilling life.

Common Symptoms

In this subchapter, we will explore some of the most common symptoms experienced by individuals with Celiac Disease. Recognizing these symptoms is crucial in managing the condition effectively and preventing further health complications. By understanding the signs of Celiac Disease, individuals can take proactive steps towards improving their overall health and well-being.

One of the most common symptoms of Celiac Disease is gastrointestinal distress. This can manifest in various ways, including abdominal pain, bloating, diarrhea, and constipation. These symptoms can be debilitating and significantly impact an individual's quality of life.

By identifying these signs early on, individuals can work towards implementing dietary and lifestyle changes that can help alleviate these symptoms and improve their digestive health.

Another common symptom of Celiac Disease is fatigue and weakness. People with Celiac Disease may experience low energy levels, even after getting an adequate amount of rest. This can be attributed to the body's inability to properly absorb essential nutrients due to damage to the small intestine.

By addressing nutritional deficiencies and following a gluten-free diet, individuals can boost their energy levels and combat feelings of fatigue.

Skin issues are also a common symptom of Celiac Disease. Individuals may experience rashes, itchiness, and dermatitis herpetiformis, a specific skin condition associated with gluten intolerance. By identifying these skin issues as potential signs of Celiac Disease, individuals can seek appropriate medical treatment and make necessary dietary changes to improve their skin health and overall well-being.

Mental health concerns, such as anxiety and depression, are also prevalent among individuals with Celiac Disease. The link between gluten intolerance and mental health issues is well-documented, and addressing these symptoms is crucial in managing the condition holistically.

By recognizing the connection between Celiac Disease and mental health, individuals can seek support from healthcare professionals, implement stress-reducing techniques, and follow a gluten-free diet to improve their overall mental well-being.

Overall, recognizing and understanding the common symptoms of Celiac Disease is essential in managing the condition effectively. By addressing gastrointestinal distress, fatigue, skin issues, and mental health concerns, individuals can take proactive steps towards improving their overall health and well-being. By adopting a holistic approach to managing Celiac Disease, individuals can enhance their quality of life and experience relief from debilitating symptoms.

How To Manage Celiac Disease Naturally

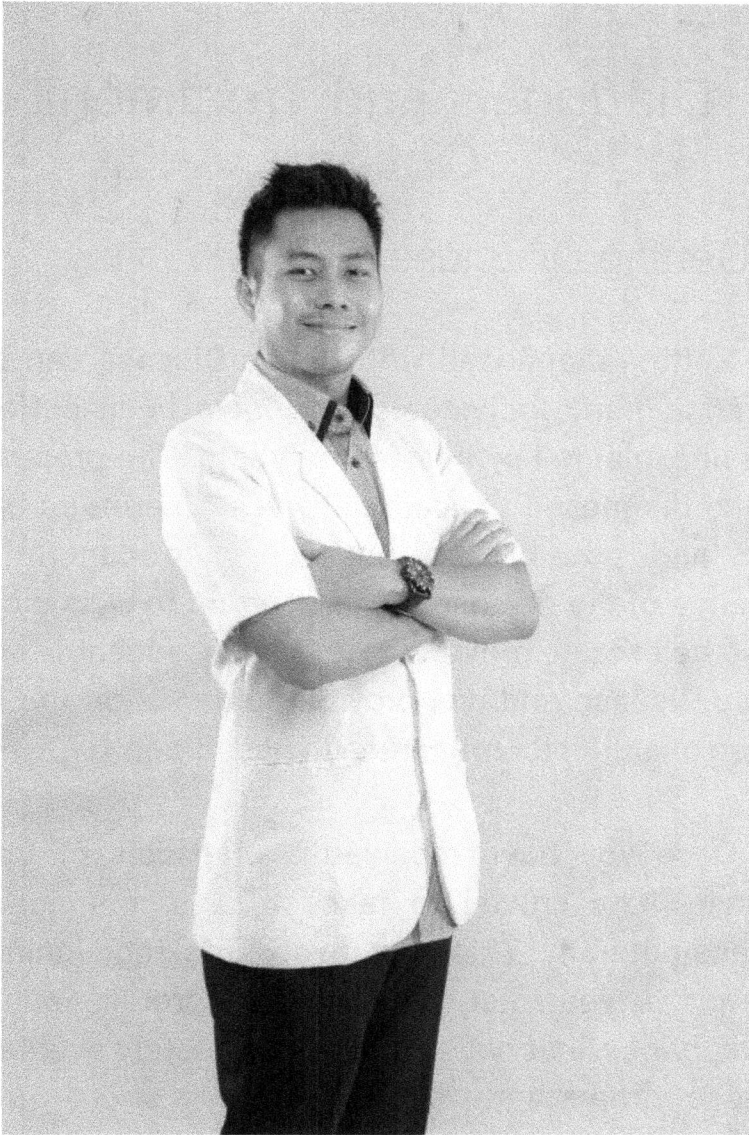

A Holistic Approach

Chapter 2

Diagnosis and Treatment Options

Getting Diagnosed

Getting diagnosed with Celiac Disease can be a relief for many individuals who have been suffering from unexplained symptoms for years. The process of getting diagnosed typically involves a series of blood tests and possibly an endoscopy to confirm the presence of the disease. It is important to work closely with a healthcare provider who is knowledgeable about Celiac Disease and can provide guidance on the best course of action for managing the condition.

Once you have received a diagnosis of Celiac Disease, it is crucial to take steps to manage the disease naturally. This may involve making significant changes to your diet, as gluten - a protein found in wheat, barley, and rye - must be completely avoided. It is also important to be vigilant about cross-contamination, as even small amounts of gluten can trigger symptoms in individuals with Celiac Disease.

In addition to dietary changes, managing Celiac Disease naturally may also involve incorporating certain supplements and herbs into your daily routine. For example, probiotics can help to support gut health and reduce inflammation, while herbs such as turmeric and ginger have anti-inflammatory properties that may help to alleviate symptoms of Celiac Disease.

It is also important to prioritize self-care when managing Celiac Disease naturally. Stress can exacerbate symptoms of the disease, so finding ways to relax and unwind, such as practicing yoga or meditation, can be beneficial. Getting regular exercise and plenty of sleep are also important for supporting overall health and managing the symptoms of Celiac Disease.

Overall, getting diagnosed with Celiac Disease can be a turning point in your health journey. By working closely with a healthcare provider and taking a holistic approach to managing the disease, you can improve your quality of life and feel better on a daily basis. Remember that you are not alone in this journey, and there are many resources available to help you navigate the challenges of living with Celiac Disease.

Medical Treatments

Medical treatments for Celiac Disease primarily involve removing gluten from your diet, as this is the only known treatment for the condition. However, there are other medical treatments that can help manage symptoms and promote healing in the body. It is important to work closely with your healthcare provider to determine the best course of treatment for you.

In addition to a gluten-free diet, some people with Celiac Disease may benefit from taking supplements to help heal the body. This can include vitamins and minerals that may be lacking due to malabsorption issues caused by the disease. Your healthcare provider can help you determine which supplements may be beneficial for you.

For some individuals with Celiac Disease, medications may be necessary to manage symptoms or complications of the condition. This can include medications to help control inflammation in the gut, as well as medications to manage other autoimmune conditions that may be present alongside Celiac Disease.

It is important to work closely with your healthcare provider to determine the best medications for your individual needs.

In addition to traditional medical treatments, there are also natural remedies that may help manage symptoms of Celiac Disease. This can include herbal supplements, acupuncture, and other holistic treatments that may help promote healing in the body. It is important to speak with your healthcare provider before beginning any new natural treatments to ensure they are safe and effective for you.

Overall, managing Celiac Disease requires a comprehensive approach that includes both medical treatments and lifestyle changes. By working closely with your healthcare provider and incorporating a gluten-free diet, supplements, medications, and natural remedies as needed, you can effectively manage your symptoms and promote healing in your body.

Remember to listen to your body and prioritize self-care to ensure you are giving yourself the best chance at managing Celiac Disease successfully.

Importance of a Gluten-Free Diet

Living with Celiac Disease can be challenging, but one of the most important steps you can take towards managing your condition naturally is adopting a gluten-free diet. Gluten is a protein found in wheat, barley, and rye that can trigger inflammation and damage the lining of the small intestine in individuals with Celiac Disease.

By eliminating gluten from your diet, you can reduce symptoms such as abdominal pain, bloating, fatigue, and nutrient deficiencies.

One of the key benefits of following a gluten-free diet is that it allows your gut to heal and repair itself. When you have Celiac Disease, consuming gluten can lead to damage to the villi in the small intestine, which are responsible for absorbing nutrients from food. By removing gluten from your diet, you can give your gut the chance to heal and improve its ability to absorb essential nutrients, leading to better overall health and well-being.

In addition to improving gut health, a gluten-free diet can also help reduce inflammation in the body. Inflammation is a common symptom of Celiac Disease and can contribute to a variety of health issues, including autoimmune conditions, joint pain, and skin problems. By avoiding gluten-containing foods, you can help decrease inflammation in your body and alleviate symptoms associated with chronic inflammation.

Following a gluten-free diet can also improve your energy levels and overall vitality. Many individuals with Celiac Disease experience fatigue and low energy levels due to malabsorption of nutrients caused by damage to the small intestine. By removing gluten from your diet and allowing your gut to heal, you may notice an increase in energy, improved concentration, and a greater sense of well-being.

Overall, adopting a gluten-free diet is essential for managing Celiac Disease naturally and promoting optimal health and wellness. By eliminating gluten-containing foods and focusing on nutrient-dense, whole foods, you can support your body's healing process, reduce inflammation, improve energy levels, and enhance your overall quality of life.

Remember to work with a healthcare provider or nutritionist to ensure you are meeting your nutritional needs while following a gluten-free diet.

How To Manage Celiac Disease Naturally

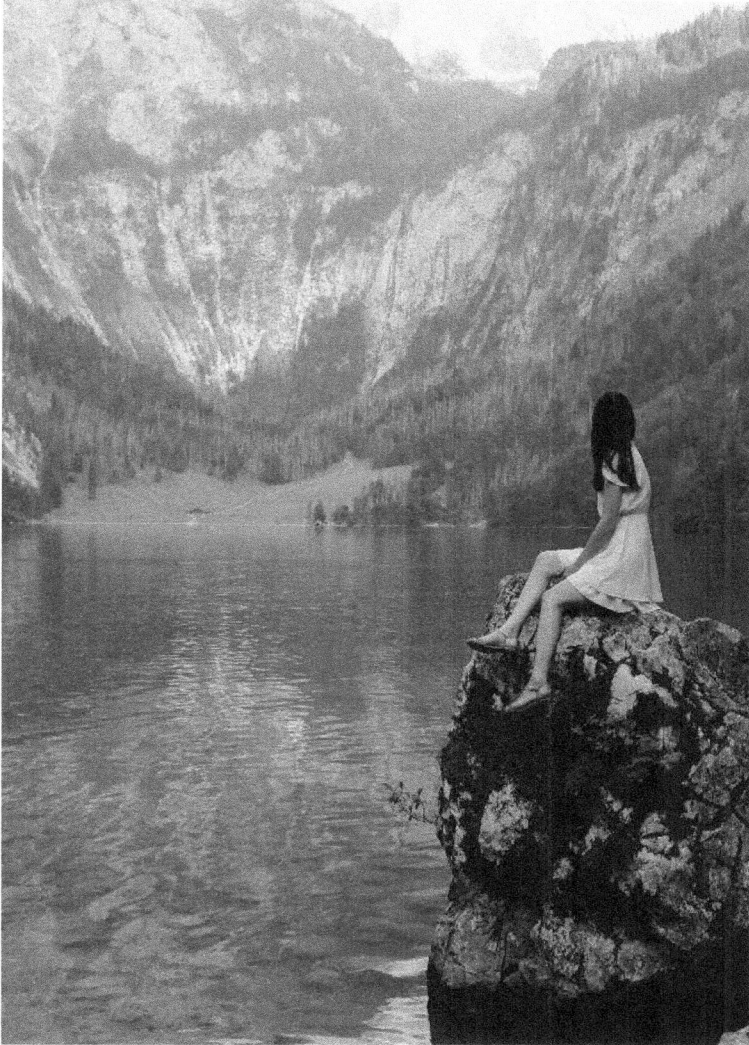

Chapter 3

The Role of Holistic Healing

Mind-Body Connection

The mind-body connection is a powerful tool for managing Celiac Disease naturally. Many people with Celiac Disease may not realize the impact that their mental and emotional state can have on their physical health. By understanding and harnessing this connection, individuals can improve their overall well-being and quality of life.

One of the key aspects of the mind-body connection is stress management. Stress has been shown to exacerbate symptoms of Celiac Disease and can even trigger flare-ups. By incorporating relaxation techniques such as deep breathing, meditation, and yoga into their daily routine, individuals can reduce stress levels and improve their overall health.

Another important component of the mind-body connection is the power of positive thinking. Research has shown that individuals who have a positive outlook on life tend to have better outcomes when managing chronic illnesses such as Celiac Disease. By focusing on the silver linings and maintaining a hopeful attitude, individuals can boost their immune system and improve their body's ability to heal.

In addition to stress management and positive thinking, maintaining a healthy lifestyle is also crucial for managing Celiac Disease naturally. This includes eating a well-balanced diet that is free from gluten, getting regular exercise, and practicing good sleep hygiene. By taking care of their physical health, individuals can support their body's natural healing processes and reduce the severity of their symptoms.

Overall, the mind-body connection is a powerful tool for managing Celiac Disease naturally. By incorporating stress management techniques, maintaining a positive attitude, and living a healthy lifestyle, individuals can improve their overall well-being and quality of life.

It is important for people with Celiac Disease to recognize the connection between their mental and physical health and to take proactive steps to support both aspects of their well-being.

Managing Stress and Anxiety

Managing stress and anxiety is crucial for individuals with Celiac Disease, as stress can exacerbate symptoms and lead to flare-ups. It is important to recognize the impact that stress and anxiety can have on the body, and take proactive steps to manage these factors in order to maintain overall health and well-being. In this chapter, we will explore various holistic approaches to managing stress and anxiety for individuals with Celiac Disease.

One effective way to manage stress and anxiety is through mindfulness and meditation practices. These techniques can help individuals with Celiac Disease to stay present in the moment, reduce racing thoughts, and promote a sense of calm and relaxation. Taking time each day to practice mindfulness can be a powerful tool in managing stress and anxiety, and can ultimately improve overall health outcomes for individuals with Celiac Disease.

In addition to mindfulness and meditation, regular exercise can also be beneficial in managing stress and anxiety for individuals with Celiac Disease. Physical activity has been shown to release endorphins, which are natural mood lifters that can help combat stress and anxiety.

Whether it's going for a walk, practicing yoga, or engaging in a favorite sport, finding ways to stay active can be an effective way to manage stress and anxiety and promote overall well-being.

Another important aspect of managing stress and anxiety for individuals with Celiac Disease is maintaining a healthy diet. Eating a well-balanced diet that is free of gluten and rich in nutrients can help to support overall physical and mental health.

Avoiding processed foods, sugar, and caffeine can also help to reduce inflammation in the body, which can contribute to stress and anxiety. By fueling the body with nourishing foods, individuals with Celiac Disease can better manage stress and anxiety and support their overall health.

Finally, it is important for individuals with Celiac Disease to prioritize self-care and relaxation techniques in their daily routine. This may include taking time for activities that bring joy and relaxation, such as reading a book, taking a bath, or spending time in nature. By incorporating self-care practices into daily life, individuals with Celiac Disease can better manage stress and anxiety, and ultimately improve their overall quality of life.

By implementing these holistic approaches to managing stress and anxiety, individuals with Celiac Disease can take proactive steps to support their physical and mental health, and ultimately thrive in their journey to healing.

Importance of Sleep

Sleep is a crucial aspect of managing celiac disease naturally. It is during sleep that our bodies repair and regenerate, allowing our immune systems to function optimally. Lack of quality sleep can lead to increased inflammation in the body, which can exacerbate symptoms of celiac disease.

It is important for individuals with celiac disease to prioritize getting enough sleep each night in order to support their overall health and well-being.

Research has shown that individuals with celiac disease who do not get enough sleep may experience more severe symptoms and longer recovery times. This is because sleep deprivation can weaken the immune system, making it more difficult for the body to fight off infections and heal damaged tissues. By prioritizing sleep, individuals with celiac disease can help their bodies recover more quickly and reduce the severity of their symptoms.

In addition to supporting immune function, adequate sleep is also important for managing stress levels. Stress can exacerbate symptoms of celiac disease and trigger flare-ups, so it is important for individuals with the condition to find ways to relax and unwind before bed. Establishing a bedtime routine, such as taking a warm bath or practicing deep breathing exercises, can help individuals with celiac disease get better quality sleep and reduce stress levels.

Furthermore, getting enough sleep can also help individuals with celiac disease maintain a healthy weight. Sleep deprivation has been linked to weight gain and obesity, both of which can worsen symptoms of celiac disease. By prioritizing sleep and maintaining a healthy weight, individuals with celiac disease can better manage their condition and improve their overall quality of life.

Overall, the importance of sleep in managing celiac disease naturally cannot be overstated. By getting enough sleep each night, individuals with celiac disease can support their immune function, reduce inflammation, manage stress levels, and maintain a healthy weight. Prioritizing sleep as part of a holistic approach to managing celiac disease can help individuals feel better, reduce symptoms, and improve their overall health and well-being.

How To Manage Celiac Disease Naturally

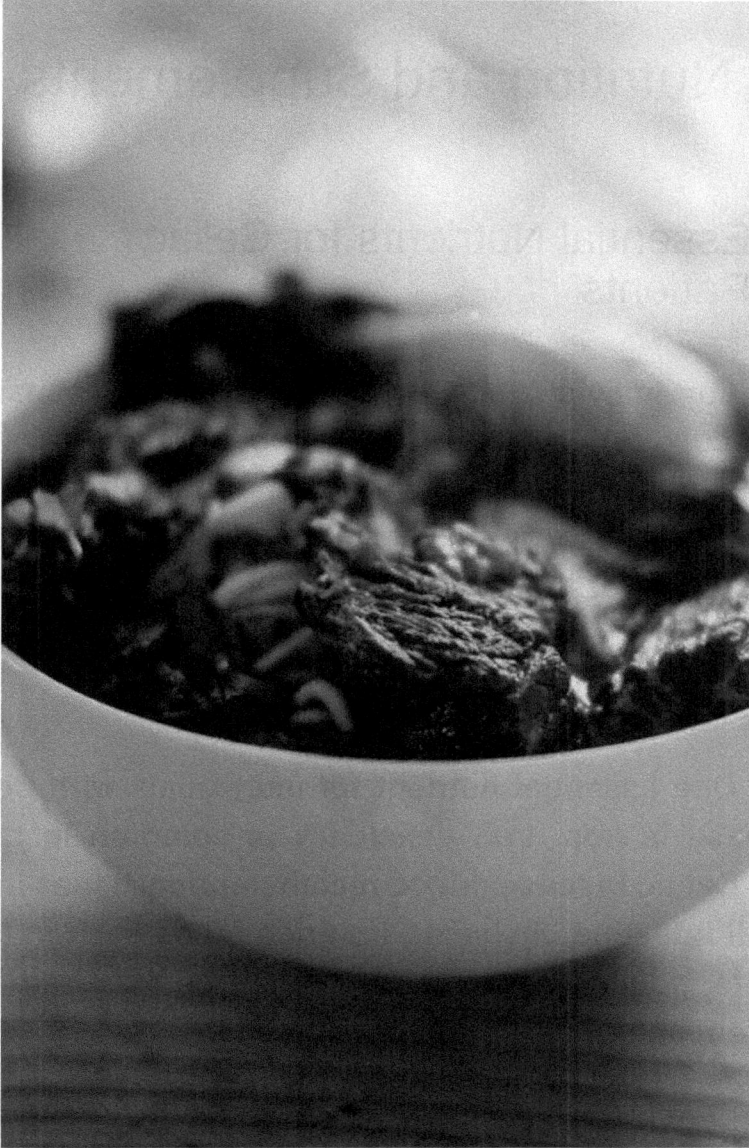

Chapter 4

Nutrition and Supplements

Essential Nutrients for Celiac Patients

For individuals with Celiac Disease, managing their condition naturally involves being mindful of the essential nutrients they need to maintain their health. In this subchapter, we will explore the key nutrients that are crucial for those with Celiac Disease to include in their diet to ensure they are getting the proper nourishment their bodies require.

One essential nutrient for individuals with Celiac Disease is iron. Iron deficiency is common in those with Celiac Disease due to malabsorption issues in the small intestine. Including iron-rich foods such as lean meats, poultry, beans, and fortified cereals can help prevent anemia and promote overall health.

Another important nutrient for Celiac patients is calcium. Since individuals with Celiac Disease may have difficulty absorbing calcium, it is important to consume foods rich in this mineral, such as dairy products, leafy greens, and fortified plant-based milks. Adequate calcium intake is essential for maintaining strong bones and teeth.

Vitamin D is also essential for those with Celiac Disease, as it plays a crucial role in bone health and immune function. Since individuals with Celiac Disease may have a higher risk of vitamin D deficiency, it is important to include sources of vitamin D in their diet, such as fatty fish, egg yolks, and fortified foods.

In addition to iron, calcium, and vitamin D, individuals with Celiac Disease should also focus on consuming foods rich in B vitamins, particularly B12 and folate. Since malabsorption can lead to deficiencies in these vitamins, incorporating sources such as lean meats, eggs, leafy greens, and fortified cereals can help prevent complications and promote optimal health.

In conclusion, ensuring a well-rounded diet that includes essential nutrients such as iron, calcium, vitamin D, and B vitamins is crucial for individuals with Celiac Disease to manage their condition naturally. By focusing on nutrient-dense foods and incorporating a variety of sources of these key nutrients, those with Celiac Disease can support their overall health and well-being.

Healing Foods for the Gut

For those who suffer from Celiac Disease, managing symptoms and promoting gut health is crucial for overall well-being. One way to support a healthy gut is through incorporating healing foods into your diet. These foods can help repair damage done to the intestines caused by gluten consumption and reduce inflammation in the gut.

One of the most beneficial healing foods for the gut is bone broth. Bone broth is rich in collagen, gelatin, and amino acids that help repair the lining of the intestines and reduce inflammation. It also contains nutrients that support overall gut health, such as glutamine, which is essential for maintaining the integrity of the intestinal barrier.

Probiotic-rich foods, such as sauerkraut, kimchi, and kefir, are also important for healing the gut. Probiotics help balance the gut microbiome and promote the growth of beneficial bacteria, which can improve digestion and reduce inflammation in the gut. Including these foods in your diet can help support a healthy gut and alleviate symptoms of Celiac Disease.

Fiber-rich foods, such as fruits, vegetables, and whole grains, are essential for promoting gut health. Fiber helps regulate digestion, support the growth of beneficial bacteria in the gut, and reduce inflammation. Including a variety of fiber-rich foods in your diet can help maintain a healthy gut and improve overall digestive health.

Incorporating healing foods for the gut into your diet is an important part of managing Celiac Disease naturally. By focusing on foods that support gut health, you can reduce inflammation, repair damage to the intestines, and alleviate symptoms of Celiac Disease. Experiment with different healing foods to find what works best for you and make them a regular part of your diet for long-term gut health.

Recommended Supplements

When managing Celiac Disease naturally, it is important to ensure that your body is receiving all the necessary nutrients it needs to heal and thrive. While a gluten-free diet is essential in managing Celiac Disease, sometimes it may not be enough to fully support your body's healing process. In these cases, incorporating certain supplements into your daily routine can be incredibly beneficial.

One of the most important supplements for people with Celiac Disease is a high-quality multivitamin. Due to the malabsorption issues that often accompany Celiac Disease, it can be difficult to get all the essential vitamins and minerals your body needs from food alone. A multivitamin can help fill in the gaps and ensure that you are getting all the nutrients necessary for optimal health.

In addition to a multivitamin, many people with Celiac Disease benefit from taking probiotics. Probiotics are essential for maintaining a healthy gut microbiome, which is crucial for overall health and immune function.

People with Celiac Disease often have imbalances in their gut flora, so taking a probiotic supplement can help restore balance and support digestion.

Another important supplement for people with Celiac Disease is vitamin D. Many people with Celiac Disease have vitamin D deficiencies, which can lead to a range of health issues. Vitamin D is essential for bone health, immune function, and overall well-being, so it is important to ensure that you are getting an adequate amount of this vital nutrient.

Omega-3 fatty acids are another important supplement for people with Celiac Disease. Omega-3s are essential for reducing inflammation in the body, which can be particularly beneficial for people with autoimmune conditions like Celiac Disease. Incorporating a high-quality omega-3 supplement into your daily routine can help support overall health and well-being.

In conclusion, while a gluten-free diet is essential for managing Celiac Disease, incorporating certain supplements into your daily routine can help support your body's healing process and overall well-being. Talk to your healthcare provider about which supplements may be right for you, and remember to choose high-quality supplements from reputable sources to ensure their effectiveness. By taking a holistic approach to managing Celiac Disease, you can support your body's healing journey and thrive in spite of your diagnosis.

How To Manage Celiac Disease Naturally

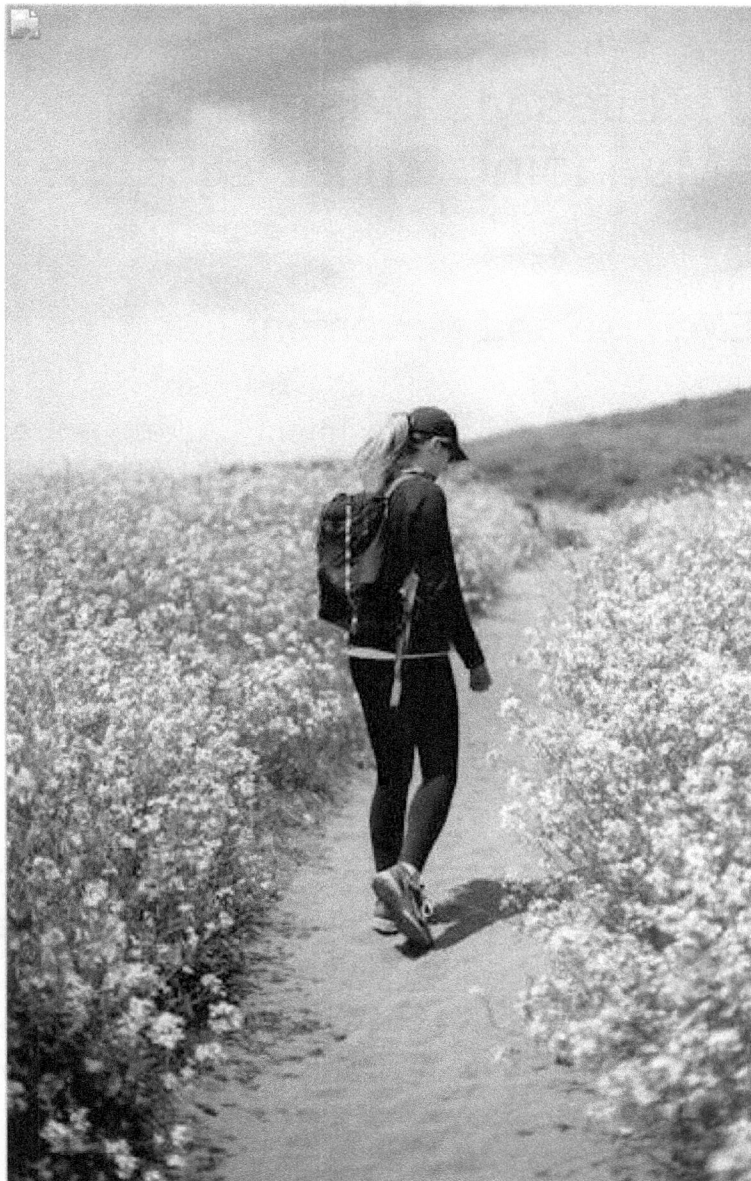

A Holistic Approach

Chapter 5

Lifestyle Changes for Managing Celiac Disease

Exercise and Movement

Exercise and movement are essential components of managing celiac disease naturally. Incorporating physical activity into your daily routine can help improve your overall health and well-being. Regular exercise can help strengthen your immune system, reduce inflammation in the body, and promote digestion and nutrient absorption, all of which are important for managing celiac disease.

There are many different types of exercises that can benefit individuals with celiac disease. Low-impact activities such as walking, swimming, and yoga are great options for those who may have limited energy or physical abilities. These exercises can help improve flexibility, balance, and strength without putting too much strain on the body.

It's important to listen to your body and choose exercises that feel good and are enjoyable for you. Remember that everyone's body is different, so what works for one person may not work for another. Experiment with different types of exercises until you find what works best for you and makes you feel good.

In addition to formal exercise routines, incorporating more movement into your daily life can also be beneficial. Simple activities like taking the stairs instead of the elevator, gardening, or playing with your children or pets can help keep you active throughout the day. The key is to find ways to incorporate movement into your daily routine that feel natural and enjoyable for you.

Overall, incorporating regular exercise and movement into your daily routine can help improve your overall health and well-being while managing celiac disease naturally. Remember to listen to your body, choose activities that feel good and are enjoyable for you, and find ways to incorporate movement into your daily life. By prioritizing exercise and movement, you can take control of your health and feel better both physically and mentally.

Social Support and Community

In the journey of managing Celiac Disease naturally, social support and community play a crucial role. Living with a chronic illness like Celiac Disease can be overwhelming at times, and having a strong support system can make all the difference.

Whether it's family, friends, or online support groups, connecting with others who understand what you're going through can provide comfort, guidance, and a sense of belonging.

One of the key benefits of social support is the emotional reassurance it can provide. Dealing with the challenges of Celiac Disease can be emotionally draining, and having a network of people who can offer empathy and understanding can help alleviate feelings of isolation and frustration.

Sharing experiences, tips, and coping strategies with others who are also managing the disease can create a sense of camaraderie and empowerment.

In addition to emotional support, social connections can also provide practical assistance. Whether it's sharing recipes, recommending safe dining options, or offering transportation to medical appointments, having a community of people who are knowledgeable about Celiac Disease can make managing the condition easier and more manageable. Knowing that you have people you can turn to for help and advice can provide a sense of security and peace of mind.

Community involvement can also be a source of motivation and inspiration. By participating in events, fundraisers, or support groups related to Celiac Disease, you can connect with others who share your journey and learn from their experiences.

Seeing how others have successfully managed the disease naturally can provide hope and encouragement, motivating you to stay committed to your own healing journey.

Overall, social support and community can be invaluable resources for individuals with Celiac Disease who are looking to manage their condition naturally. By building connections with others who understand and support you, you can find comfort, guidance, and motivation to navigate the challenges of living with a chronic illness. Remember, you are not alone in this journey, and there are people who are ready and willing to help you every step of the way.

Managing Cross-Contamination

Managing cross-contamination is a crucial aspect of living with celiac disease. Even a small amount of gluten can trigger symptoms and damage the intestines of someone with celiac disease. It is important to be vigilant in order to prevent cross-contamination and maintain a gluten-free lifestyle. Here are some tips on how to manage cross-contamination effectively.

First and foremost, it is important to educate yourself about sources of gluten and how cross-contamination can occur. Gluten can be found in a wide variety of products, including processed foods, condiments, and even medications.

Cross-contamination can happen in the kitchen, at restaurants, or even when dining with friends or family. By understanding these risks, you can take proactive steps to minimize them.

One of the most important steps in managing cross-contamination is to create a dedicated gluten-free kitchen. This means keeping separate utensils, cookware, and food storage containers for gluten-free items. It is also important to thoroughly clean surfaces, such as countertops and cutting boards, to prevent any traces of gluten from contaminating your food. By creating a safe space in your kitchen, you can reduce the risk of accidental exposure to gluten.

When dining out or attending social events, it is important to communicate your dietary needs clearly. Make sure to ask about ingredients and how dishes are prepared to ensure they are gluten-free. It may also be helpful to bring your own food or snacks to events to avoid potential cross-contamination. By advocating for yourself and being proactive about your needs, you can reduce the risk of accidental exposure to gluten.

In addition to being vigilant about your food choices, it is important to also be mindful of other sources of gluten. This includes personal care products, such as shampoo, lotion, and toothpaste, which can contain hidden sources of gluten. By reading labels and choosing gluten-free products, you can protect yourself from potential cross-contamination. It may also be helpful to educate those around you, such as family members and caregivers, about the importance of avoiding gluten in all forms.

Managing cross-contamination requires diligence and awareness, but it is possible to live a healthy and fulfilling life with celiac disease. By taking proactive steps to prevent exposure to gluten, you can protect your health and well-being. Remember to stay informed, communicate your needs clearly, and advocate for yourself in all situations. With the right strategies in place, you can successfully manage cross-contamination and enjoy a gluten-free lifestyle.

How To Manage Celiac Disease Naturally

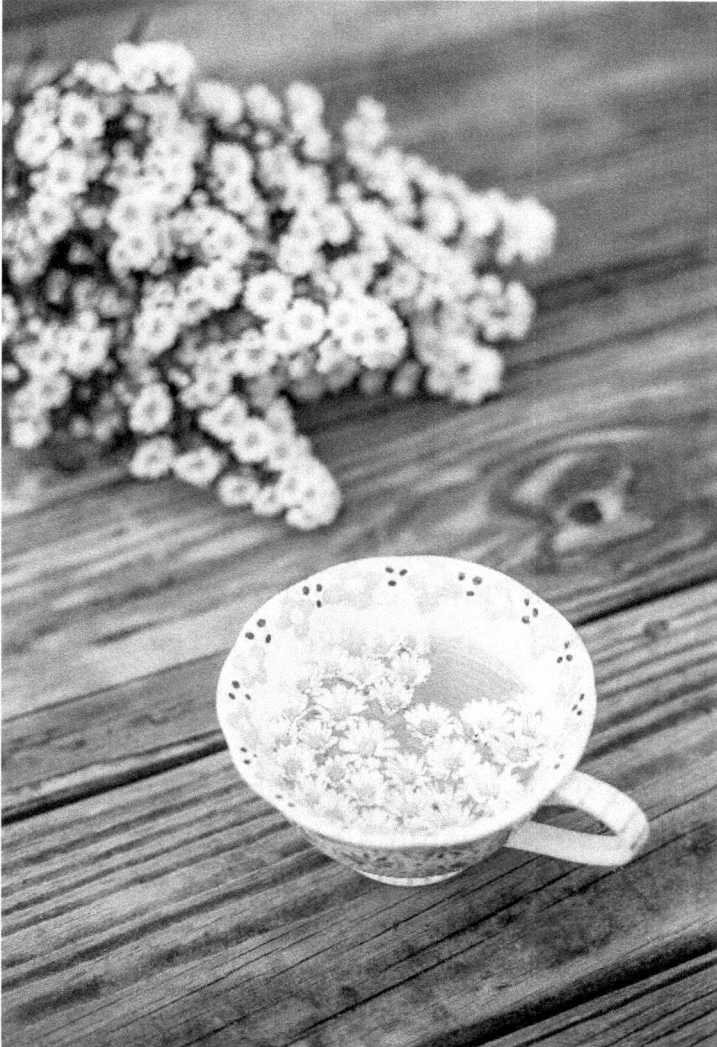

Chapter 6

Holistic Approaches to Healing

Herbal Remedies and Alternative Therapies

Living with Celiac Disease can be challenging, but there are many natural remedies and alternative therapies that can help manage symptoms and improve overall well-being. Herbal remedies have been used for centuries to treat a variety of ailments, including digestive issues like those associated with Celiac Disease. Some popular herbs for managing Celiac symptoms include ginger, peppermint, and chamomile. These herbs can help soothe an upset stomach, reduce inflammation in the gut, and aid in digestion.

In addition to herbal remedies, there are several alternative therapies that can be beneficial for those with Celiac Disease.

Acupuncture, for example, has been shown to reduce pain and inflammation in the body, which can be especially helpful for those experiencing gastrointestinal discomfort. Massage therapy is another alternative therapy that can help relax the muscles in the abdomen and improve digestion. Yoga and meditation are also great practices for managing stress, which can exacerbate Celiac symptoms.

It's important to remember that while herbal remedies and alternative therapies can be helpful in managing Celiac Disease, they are not a substitute for a gluten-free diet. The only way to effectively manage Celiac Disease is to completely eliminate gluten from your diet. However, incorporating herbal remedies and alternative therapies can help alleviate symptoms and improve overall quality of life for those with the disease.

Before incorporating any new herbal remedies or alternative therapies into your routine, it's important to consult with a healthcare professional or holistic practitioner. They can help determine which remedies are safe and effective for you based on your individual needs and health history.

It's also important to remember that what works for one person may not work for another, so it may take some trial and error to find the right combination of remedies that work best for you.

Overall, taking a holistic approach to managing Celiac Disease, including incorporating herbal remedies and alternative therapies, can help improve symptoms and quality of life for those with the disease. By combining these natural treatments with a gluten-free diet and regular medical care, individuals with Celiac Disease can take control of their health and well-being in a comprehensive and effective way.

Mindfulness and Meditation Practices

Mindfulness and meditation practices are powerful tools that can greatly benefit individuals with Celiac Disease. By incorporating these practices into your daily routine, you can reduce stress, improve mental clarity, and enhance overall well-being. Mindfulness involves being fully present in the moment, without judgment or attachment to thoughts or emotions.

This can help you better cope with the challenges of living with Celiac Disease, such as managing symptoms, navigating social situations, and maintaining a gluten-free diet.

One way to practice mindfulness is through meditation. Meditation involves focusing your attention on your breath, a mantra, or a particular sensation, in order to cultivate a sense of inner peace and calm. By regularly engaging in meditation, you can train your mind to be more present and aware, which can help you better manage the stress and anxiety that often accompany Celiac Disease.

Meditation can also help you develop a greater sense of self-awareness and compassion, which can be particularly beneficial when dealing with the physical and emotional challenges of living with a chronic illness.

In addition to meditation, there are many other mindfulness practices that can benefit individuals with Celiac Disease. These may include yoga, tai chi, qigong, or simply taking time each day to engage in activities that bring you joy and relaxation.

By incorporating these practices into your daily routine, you can cultivate a greater sense of balance and well-being, which can help you better manage your symptoms and improve your overall quality of life.

It is important to remember that mindfulness and meditation are not quick fixes, but rather long-term practices that require commitment and dedication. It may take time to see the full benefits of these practices, but with consistent effort, you can experience profound changes in your mental, emotional, and physical health.

By incorporating mindfulness and meditation into your daily routine, you can cultivate a greater sense of peace, resilience, and acceptance, which can greatly enhance your ability to manage Celiac Disease naturally and holistically.

In conclusion, mindfulness and meditation practices are powerful tools that can greatly benefit individuals with Celiac Disease. By incorporating these practices into your daily routine, you can reduce stress, improve mental clarity, and enhance overall well-being.

Remember that these practices require commitment and dedication, but with consistent effort, you can experience profound changes in your mental, emotional, and physical health. Embrace mindfulness and meditation as essential components of your holistic approach to managing Celiac Disease naturally.

Energy Healing Modalities

Energy healing modalities are alternative therapies that focus on the body's energy systems to promote healing and balance. For those living with Celiac Disease, these modalities can be a valuable addition to their holistic approach to managing their condition. By working with the body's energy fields, energy healing modalities can help to alleviate symptoms, reduce inflammation, and support overall well-being.

One popular energy healing modality for those with Celiac Disease is Reiki. Reiki is a Japanese technique that uses the practitioner's hands to channel energy into the body to promote relaxation and healing.

By balancing the body's energy systems, Reiki can help to reduce stress, boost the immune system, and improve digestion - all of which are important factors in managing Celiac Disease.

Another energy healing modality that can benefit those with Celiac Disease is acupuncture. Acupuncture is a traditional Chinese medicine practice that involves inserting thin needles into specific points on the body to promote energy flow and balance. For individuals with Celiac Disease, acupuncture can help to reduce inflammation, alleviate digestive issues, and improve overall energy levels.

Crystals and gemstones are another energy healing modality that can be beneficial for those with Celiac Disease. Certain crystals, such as amethyst and citrine, are believed to have healing properties that can help to balance the body's energy systems and promote overall well-being. By incorporating crystals into their daily routine, individuals with Celiac Disease can enhance their healing process and support their body's natural ability to heal.

Sound healing is another energy healing modality that can be beneficial for those with Celiac Disease. Sound therapy involves using sound frequencies, such as singing bowls or tuning forks, to promote relaxation, reduce stress, and improve overall well-being. By incorporating sound healing into their self-care routine, individuals with Celiac Disease can support their body's healing process and promote a sense of balance and harmony.

How To Manage Celiac Disease Naturally

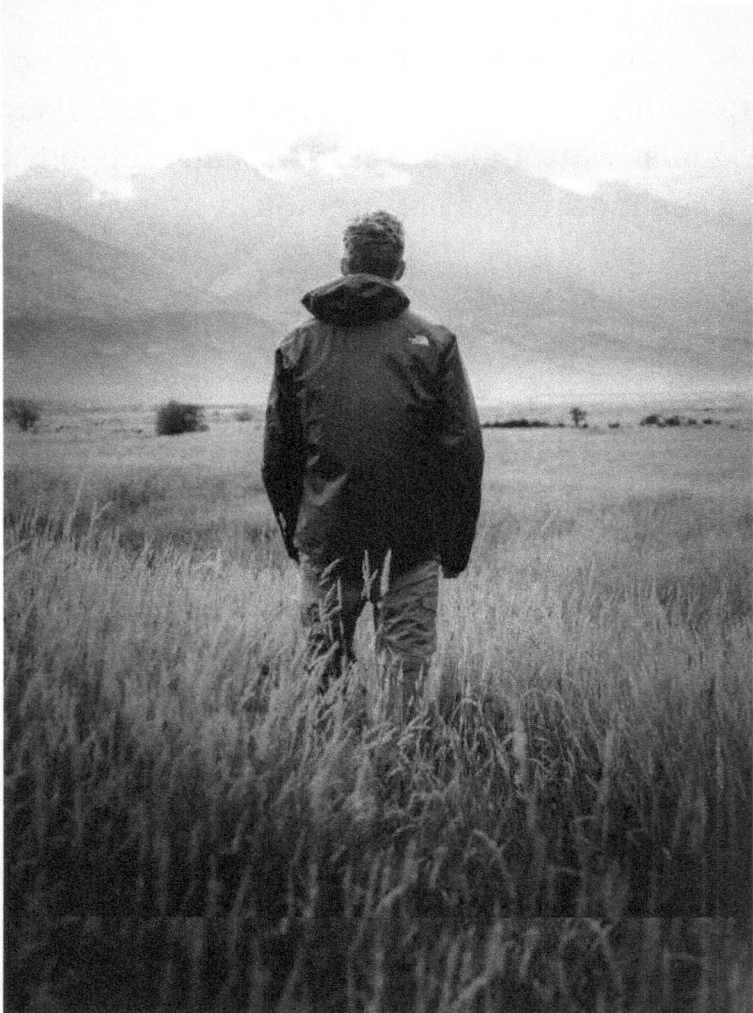

A Holistic Approach

Chapter 7

Creating a Personalized Healing Plan

Setting Goals and Intentions

Setting goals and intentions is a crucial step in managing Celiac Disease naturally. By setting clear and achievable goals, individuals with Celiac Disease can take control of their health and well-being. It is important to establish goals that are specific, measurable, attainable, relevant, and time-bound (SMART). By doing so, individuals can track their progress and stay motivated on their healing journey.

One goal that individuals with Celiac Disease may want to set is to focus on healing their gut. This can be done through a combination of dietary changes, supplements, and lifestyle modifications. By setting the intention to prioritize gut health, individuals can work towards reducing inflammation, improving digestion, and enhancing nutrient absorption. This can help to alleviate symptoms of Celiac Disease and promote overall wellness.

Another important goal for individuals with Celiac Disease is to educate themselves about the condition and how to manage it effectively. By setting the intention to learn about gluten-free living, reading up on the latest research, and seeking guidance from healthcare professionals, individuals can become empowered to make informed decisions about their health. This can lead to better treatment outcomes and a higher quality of life.

Setting goals and intentions can also help individuals with Celiac Disease to stay on track with their gluten-free diet.

By establishing a meal plan, setting aside time for meal prep, and creating a supportive environment at home, individuals can make it easier to stick to their dietary restrictions. By setting the intention to prioritize their health and well-being, individuals can overcome challenges and temptations that may arise.

In conclusion, setting goals and intentions is a powerful tool for individuals with Celiac Disease to take control of their health and well-being.

By establishing clear and achievable goals, focusing on healing the gut, educating themselves about the condition, and staying on track with their gluten-free diet, individuals can manage Celiac Disease naturally and improve their quality of life. By setting the intention to prioritize their health, individuals can overcome obstacles and achieve lasting healing.

Tracking Progress and Adjusting Strategies

As you embark on your journey to manage Celiac Disease naturally, it is important to track your progress and adjust your strategies accordingly. Monitoring your symptoms, diet, and overall well-being can provide valuable insights into what is working and what may need to be modified in your approach to healing.

One way to track your progress is to keep a detailed journal of your daily experiences. Note any changes in your symptoms, energy levels, and mood, as well as any new foods or supplements you have introduced into your diet.

By documenting these factors, you can begin to identify patterns and correlations that may help you better understand how your body reacts to certain stimuli.

In addition to keeping a journal, it can be helpful to work with a healthcare provider who is knowledgeable about Celiac Disease and natural healing methods. They can help you interpret your journal entries, recommend adjustments to your diet or lifestyle, and provide guidance on incorporating holistic practices such as acupuncture, herbal medicine, or mindfulness techniques into your treatment plan.

When tracking your progress, it is also important to be patient and realistic about your expectations. Healing Celiac Disease naturally is a process that takes time and dedication, and results may not be immediate. By staying committed to your health goals and making gradual, sustainable changes to your lifestyle, you can set yourself up for long-term success in managing your condition.

Remember that managing Celiac Disease naturally is a journey, not a destination. By tracking your progress, adjusting your strategies as needed, and staying connected to your body and healthcare team, you can empower yourself to take control of your health and live a vibrant, fulfilling life despite the challenges of this autoimmune condition.

Maintaining a Positive Mindset

Maintaining a positive mindset is crucial when managing Celiac Disease naturally. Living with a chronic illness can be challenging, but it is important to remember that a positive attitude can greatly impact your overall well-being. By focusing on the things you can control and finding ways to stay positive, you can better manage your symptoms and improve your quality of life.

One way to maintain a positive mindset is to practice gratitude. Take time each day to reflect on the things you are grateful for, whether it's the support of loved ones, a beautiful sunset, or a delicious gluten-free meal.

Cultivating a sense of gratitude can help shift your focus away from the challenges of living with Celiac Disease and towards the positive aspects of your life.

Another important aspect of maintaining a positive mindset is self-care. Taking care of yourself both physically and emotionally is essential when managing a chronic illness like Celiac Disease. Make sure to prioritize activities that bring you joy and relaxation, such as spending time outdoors, practicing yoga, or indulging in a hobby you love. By taking care of yourself, you can better cope with the challenges of living with Celiac Disease.

It is also important to surround yourself with a supportive community. Connecting with others who understand what you are going through can provide a sense of comfort and belonging. Consider joining a support group for people with Celiac Disease, or reaching out to friends and family members who can offer support and understanding. Having a strong support system can help you stay positive and motivated on your journey to managing Celiac Disease naturally.

Lastly, remember to be kind to yourself. Living with a chronic illness can be tough, and it's important to treat yourself with compassion and understanding. If you have a setback or a bad day, don't be too hard on yourself. Instead, practice self-compassion and remind yourself that you are doing the best you can. By maintaining a positive mindset and treating yourself with kindness, you can better navigate the challenges of living with Celiac Disease and improve your overall well-being.

How To Manage Celiac Disease Naturally

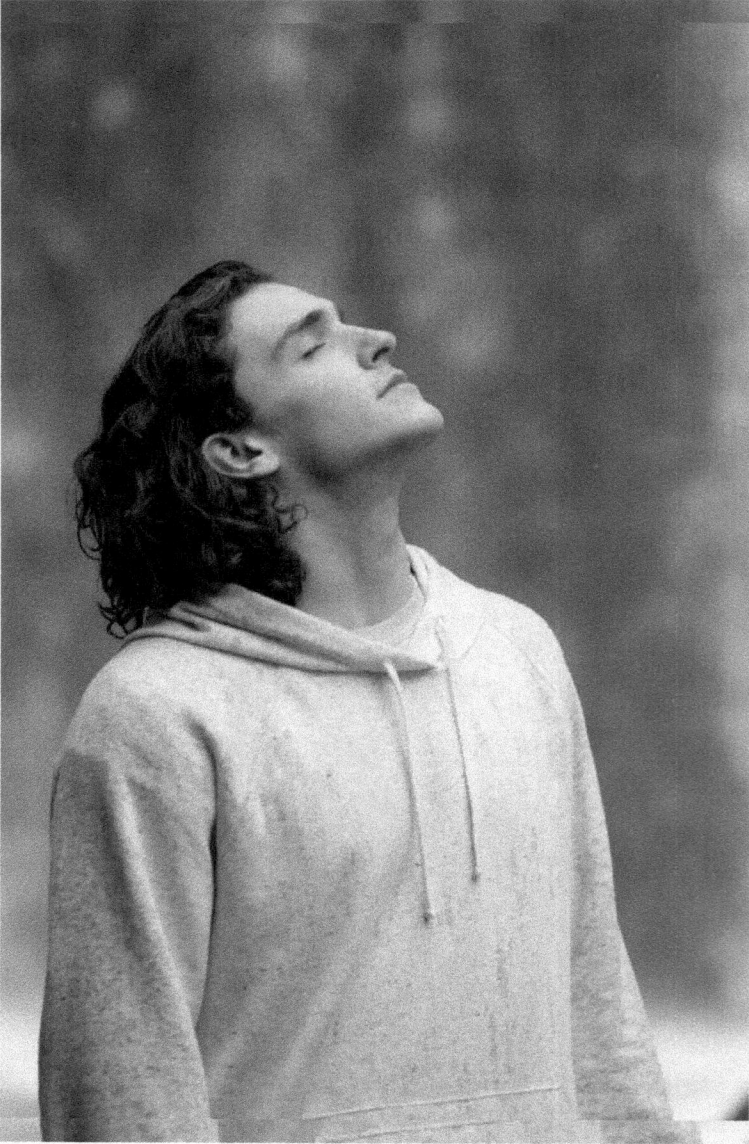

A Holistic Approach

Chapter 8

Navigating Challenges and Setbacks

Dealing with Food Cravings

Dealing with food cravings can be a challenging aspect of managing Celiac Disease, as many of the foods that people crave may contain gluten. However, it is important to remember that there are plenty of delicious gluten-free alternatives available that can satisfy your cravings without compromising your health. By being mindful of your cravings and making conscious decisions about what you eat, you can navigate this aspect of living with Celiac Disease successfully.

One strategy for dealing with food cravings is to identify the underlying cause of the craving. Are you craving something sweet because you are stressed or tired? Are you craving something salty because you are dehydrated? By understanding the root cause of your cravings, you can address the underlying issue rather than simply trying to suppress the craving with unhealthy foods.

Another tip for managing food cravings is to stock your kitchen with plenty of gluten-free snacks and treats that you enjoy. This way, when a craving strikes, you have a healthy option readily available. Keep a variety of gluten-free snacks on hand, such as nuts, seeds, fruit, and gluten-free crackers, so that you always have something to reach for when a craving hits.

It can also be helpful to plan your meals and snacks in advance to prevent cravings from taking over. By having a meal plan in place, you can ensure that you are getting all of the nutrients you need and avoid the temptation of reaching for unhealthy foods when hunger strikes. Make sure to include plenty of protein, fiber, and healthy fats in your meals to help keep you satisfied and prevent cravings.

Lastly, practicing mindfulness and self-care can also be beneficial in managing food cravings. Take time to relax and de-stress, as cravings can often be triggered by emotional factors. Engage in activities that bring you joy and fulfillment, such as yoga, meditation, or spending time with loved ones.

By taking care of your mental and emotional well-being, you can better manage your cravings and make healthy choices that support your overall health and well-being.

Coping with Social Situations

Coping with social situations can be one of the biggest challenges for people with Celiac Disease. Whether you're attending a family gathering, going out to eat with friends, or attending a work function, the fear of accidentally ingesting gluten can be overwhelming. However, there are ways to navigate these situations with confidence and ease.

One of the best ways to cope with social situations is to be prepared. Before attending an event, reach out to the host or restaurant ahead of time to discuss your dietary needs. This way, they can accommodate your needs and you can feel more at ease knowing that there will be safe options for you to eat. Additionally, consider bringing your own gluten-free snacks or dishes to share with others, so you know there will be something safe for you to eat.

Another important aspect of coping with social situations is communication. Don't be afraid to speak up about your dietary restrictions and needs. Educate those around you about Celiac Disease and how important it is for you to avoid gluten.

By being open and honest about your condition, you can help others understand and support you in making safe food choices.

In social situations where you may not have control over the food being served, such as at a potluck or restaurant, it's crucial to be vigilant about reading labels and asking questions about ingredients. Don't be afraid to inquire about how the food was prepared and if there is any risk of cross-contamination. It's better to be safe than sorry when it comes to your health.

Lastly, remember that it's okay to prioritize your health and well-being in social situations. If you're uncomfortable or unsure about the food being served, it's okay to politely decline and eat beforehand or bring your own meal.

Your health is the most important thing, and there's no shame in taking care of yourself. By being proactive, communicative, and assertive in social situations, you can navigate them with confidence and ease while managing your Celiac Disease naturally.

Overcoming Plateaus in Healing

Healing from Celiac Disease is a journey that can be filled with ups and downs. It is common for individuals to experience plateaus in their healing process, where progress seems to stall or even regress. However, it is important to remember that these plateaus are a natural part of the healing process and can be overcome with patience and perseverance.

One of the keys to overcoming plateaus in healing from Celiac Disease is to maintain a holistic approach to managing the condition. This means addressing not only the physical symptoms of the disease, but also the emotional and mental aspects that can impact overall health. Incorporating stress-reducing practices such as meditation, yoga, or deep breathing exercises can help to support the body's healing process and break through plateaus.

Another important aspect of overcoming plateaus in healing is to regularly reassess and adjust your treatment plan. As the body heals, its needs may change, requiring modifications to your diet, supplements, or other healing modalities. Working closely with a holistic healthcare provider who understands Celiac Disease and its impact on the body can help to ensure that your treatment plan is tailored to your individual needs and goals.

It is also important to remember that healing from Celiac Disease is not a linear process. There may be times when progress seems slow or non-existent, but this does not mean that you are not making progress. Trust in your body's innate ability to heal and know that with time and persistence, you can overcome plateaus and continue on your journey towards optimal health.

In conclusion, overcoming plateaus in healing from Celiac Disease requires a holistic approach, regular reassessment of your treatment plan, and trust in your body's ability to heal. By incorporating stress-reducing practices, working closely with a healthcare provider, and staying committed to your healing journey, you can break through plateaus and continue on the path towards vibrant health and well-being.

How To Manage Celiac Disease Naturally

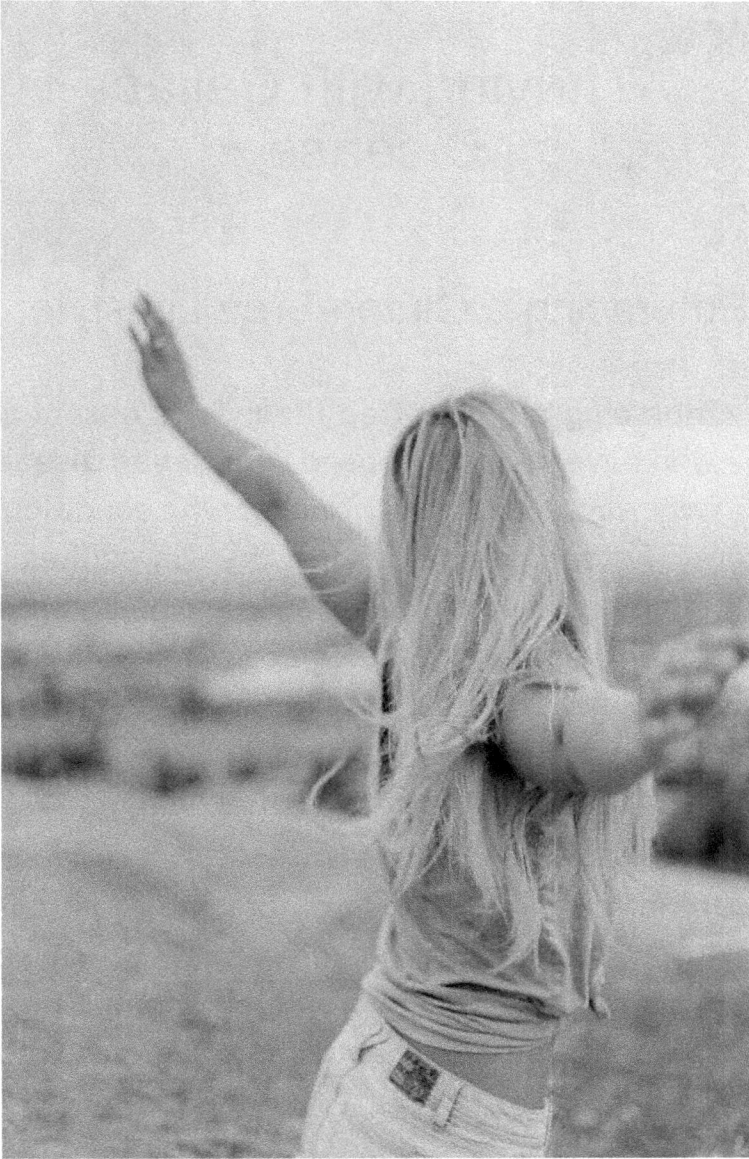

A Holistic Approach

Chapter 9

Thriving with Celiac Disease

Embracing a Gluten-Free Lifestyle

Embracing a gluten-free lifestyle is essential for those who have been diagnosed with Celiac Disease. It is the only way to effectively manage the condition and prevent further damage to the intestines. By eliminating gluten from your diet, you can significantly reduce symptoms such as stomach pain, bloating, and fatigue. It may seem daunting at first, but with the right resources and support, transitioning to a gluten-free lifestyle can be empowering and life-changing.

One of the first steps in embracing a gluten-free lifestyle is educating yourself about which foods contain gluten and which are safe to eat. Gluten is found in wheat, barley, rye, and many processed foods.

It is important to read labels carefully and be aware of hidden sources of gluten in ingredients such as modified food starch, malt extract, and soy sauce. By familiarizing yourself with gluten-free alternatives and cooking techniques, you can confidently navigate grocery shopping and meal preparation.

In addition to eliminating gluten from your diet, it is important to focus on incorporating nutrient-dense foods that support gut health and overall well-being. Foods such as fruits, vegetables, lean proteins, and gluten-free whole grains can provide essential vitamins, minerals, and antioxidants that promote healing and reduce inflammation in the body. Experimenting with new recipes and exploring different cuisines can make the gluten-free lifestyle more enjoyable and sustainable in the long run.

Managing stress and practicing self-care are also key components of embracing a gluten-free lifestyle. Stress can exacerbate symptoms of Celiac Disease and hinder the healing process. Engaging in relaxation techniques such as meditation, yoga, and deep breathing exercises can help reduce stress levels and improve overall health.

Making time for hobbies, socializing with loved ones, and getting regular exercise are important for maintaining a balanced and fulfilling lifestyle while managing Celiac Disease naturally.

Ultimately, embracing a gluten-free lifestyle is a journey of self-discovery and empowerment. By taking control of your health and making informed choices about your diet and lifestyle, you can not only manage Celiac Disease effectively but also thrive and live a vibrant, fulfilling life. Remember that you are not alone in this journey, and there are resources and support systems available to help you every step of the way. Stay positive, stay informed, and stay committed to your health and well-being.

Finding Joy and Fulfillment

Living with Celiac Disease can be challenging, but it doesn't have to define your life. In fact, finding joy and fulfillment is not only possible, but essential for managing the disease naturally. By focusing on self-care, positive thinking, and making small changes to your lifestyle, you can improve your overall well-being and quality of life.

One of the first steps to finding joy and fulfillment with Celiac Disease is to prioritize self-care. This means taking the time to nourish your body with nutrient-dense foods that support your immune system and digestive health.

It also means making time for activities that bring you joy and relaxation, such as yoga, meditation, or spending time in nature. By taking care of yourself physically, emotionally, and mentally, you can better manage the symptoms of Celiac Disease and improve your overall quality of life.

Positive thinking is another key component of finding joy and fulfillment with Celiac Disease. It's easy to get caught up in negative thoughts and feelings when dealing with a chronic illness, but focusing on the positive aspects of your life can help shift your mindset and improve your overall well-being.

By practicing gratitude, mindfulness, and self-compassion, you can cultivate a more positive outlook and find joy in the present moment, despite the challenges of living with Celiac Disease.

Making small changes to your lifestyle can also help you find joy and fulfillment with Celiac Disease. This might include finding new gluten-free recipes to enjoy, exploring new hobbies or interests, or connecting with others who share similar experiences. By embracing these changes and seeking out new opportunities for growth and connection, you can create a more fulfilling life that is centered around your health and well-being.

In conclusion, finding joy and fulfillment with Celiac Disease is not only possible, but essential for managing the disease naturally. By prioritizing self-care, cultivating positive thinking, and making small changes to your lifestyle, you can improve your overall quality of life and find joy in the present moment.

Remember that you are not defined by your illness, and that you have the power to create a life that is fulfilling, vibrant, and joyful, despite the challenges of living with Celiac Disease.

Inspiring Others on the Healing Journey

When you are on the healing journey of managing Celiac Disease naturally, it is important to remember that you are not alone. There are many others who have walked this path before you and have found success in improving their health and well-being.

By sharing your own story and experiences, you can inspire others who may be struggling with the challenges of living with Celiac Disease.

One way to inspire others on the healing journey is to lead by example. By showing how you have made positive changes in your life to manage your Celiac Disease naturally, you can motivate others to do the same.

Whether it is through sharing your favorite gluten-free recipes, tips for navigating social situations, or strategies for dealing with symptoms, your personal journey can serve as a source of inspiration for others.

Another way to inspire others on the healing journey is to offer support and encouragement. Living with Celiac Disease can be challenging, especially when faced with social pressures, dietary restrictions, and potential health complications.

By connecting with others who are also managing their Celiac Disease naturally, you can provide a sense of community and understanding that can help others feel less alone in their struggles.

Sharing success stories and celebrating milestones can also be a powerful way to inspire others on the healing journey. Whether it is reaching a health goal, overcoming a dietary challenge, or simply feeling better overall, highlighting the positive aspects of managing Celiac Disease naturally can motivate others to continue on their own path to healing.

By acknowledging and celebrating the progress that has been made, you can inspire others to keep moving forward in their own journey.

In the end, inspiring others on the healing journey is about sharing your knowledge, experiences, and support in a way that empowers others to take control of their health and well-being. By being a source of inspiration and encouragement, you can help others see that managing Celiac Disease naturally is not only possible but can also lead to a happier and healthier life. Remember, we are all in this together, and by lifting each other up, we can make the journey to healing a little bit easier for everyone.

How To Manage Celiac Disease Naturally

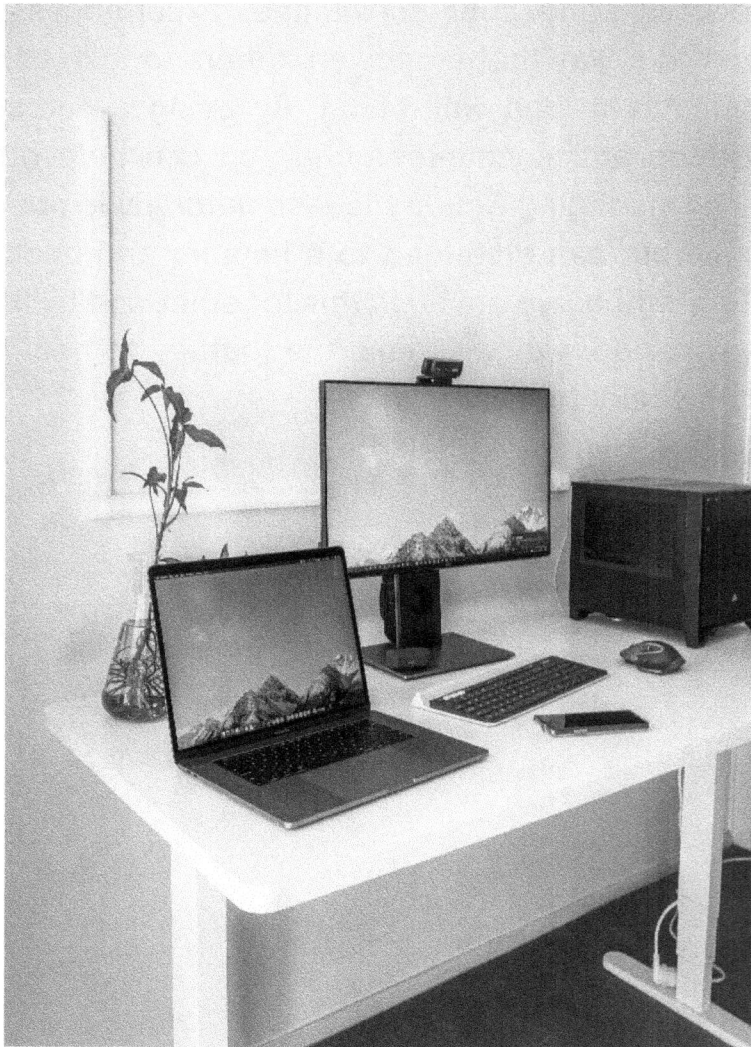

A Holistic Approach

Chapter 10

Resources for Continued Support

Support Groups and Online Communities

Support groups and online communities can be invaluable resources for individuals living with Celiac Disease. These groups provide a platform for people to connect with others who are facing similar challenges and can offer a sense of community and understanding that may be lacking in their day-to-day lives. By sharing experiences, advice, and information, members of these groups can support each other in managing their condition and navigating the complexities of living a gluten-free lifestyle.

One of the key benefits of participating in a support group or online community is the opportunity to learn from others who have successfully managed their Celiac Disease naturally.

Members can share tips on finding safe and delicious gluten-free foods, coping with social situations, and dealing with the emotional and psychological aspects of living with a chronic illness. This peer support can be incredibly empowering and can help individuals feel less isolated and more empowered in their journey towards better health.

In addition to emotional support, support groups and online communities can also provide valuable practical advice and resources. Members can exchange information on gluten-free recipes, product recommendations, and strategies for dining out safely. They can also share updates on the latest research and developments in the field of Celiac Disease, ensuring that everyone stays informed and up-to-date on the best practices for managing their condition naturally.

For many individuals with Celiac Disease, finding a supportive and understanding community can be a game-changer in their journey towards healing. Support groups and online communities offer a safe space for individuals to ask questions, seek advice, and share their struggles and triumphs with others who truly understand what they are going through.

By connecting with like-minded individuals, people with Celiac Disease can gain a sense of validation, empowerment, and hope for the future.

In conclusion, support groups and online communities can play a crucial role in helping individuals with Celiac Disease manage their condition naturally. By providing emotional support, practical advice, and a sense of community, these groups can empower individuals to take control of their health and well-being. For anyone living with Celiac Disease, joining a support group or online community can be a powerful step towards healing and living a fulfilling life free from gluten.

Recommended Books and Websites

For individuals looking to manage their Celiac Disease naturally, there are a plethora of resources available in the form of books and websites that provide valuable information and guidance. These resources can help you understand the condition better and provide practical tips on how to navigate the challenges of living with Celiac Disease.

Here are some recommended books and websites that can serve as valuable tools in your journey towards healing:

One highly recommended book for individuals with Celiac Disease is "The Gluten-Free Bible" by Jax Peters Lowell. This comprehensive guide provides practical advice on living a gluten-free lifestyle, including tips on how to navigate social situations, dining out, and cooking at home. Lowell shares her own personal experiences with Celiac Disease, making this book a relatable and informative resource for those looking to manage their condition naturally.

Another excellent resource for individuals with Celiac Disease is the website Gluten-Free Living (glutenfreeliving.com). This website offers a wealth of information on gluten-free living, including recipes, product reviews, and tips for managing Celiac Disease. The website also features articles written by experts in the field, providing valuable insights into the latest research and developments in the world of gluten-free living.

For individuals looking to take a holistic approach to managing their Celiac Disease, the book "Healing Celiac Disease Naturally" by Jessica Black, N.D. is a must-read. This book explores the connection between diet, lifestyle, and overall health, offering practical advice on how to support your body's natural healing process.

Black emphasizes the importance of a whole foods diet, stress management, and self-care practices as key components of managing Celiac Disease naturally.

In addition to books and websites, support groups can also be valuable resources for individuals with Celiac Disease. Websites such as Beyond Celiac (beyondceliac.org) and the Celiac Disease Foundation (celiac.org) offer information on local support groups, online forums, and resources for individuals looking to connect with others who are living with Celiac Disease.

These support groups can provide valuable emotional support, practical advice, and a sense of community for individuals navigating the challenges of managing Celiac Disease naturally.

Overall, books and websites can be valuable tools for individuals looking to manage their Celiac Disease naturally. By educating yourself, connecting with others, and exploring holistic approaches to healing, you can empower yourself to take control of your health and well-being. Remember, you are not alone in your journey – there are resources and support available to help you live a healthy, fulfilling life with Celiac Disease.

Finding Holistic Practitioners and Healthcare Providers

Finding holistic practitioners and healthcare providers who understand and support your journey with Celiac Disease is essential for managing your condition naturally. These practitioners take a whole-body approach to health, focusing on the interconnectedness of physical, mental, emotional, and spiritual well-being. When seeking out holistic practitioners, look for those who have experience working with individuals with Celiac Disease and who are open to integrating complementary and alternative treatments into your care plan.

One way to find holistic practitioners and healthcare providers is to ask for referrals from other individuals with Celiac Disease who have had positive experiences. You can also search online directories, such as the Institute for Functional Medicine or the American Holistic Medical Association, to find practitioners in your area. Additionally, consider reaching out to local health food stores, yoga studios, or wellness centers for recommendations on holistic practitioners who specialize in treating autoimmune conditions like Celiac Disease.

When meeting with a potential holistic practitioner or healthcare provider, be sure to ask about their experience working with individuals with Celiac Disease and inquire about their approach to treatment. Look for practitioners who are knowledgeable about the role of diet, stress management, and gut health in managing Celiac Disease symptoms.

Additionally, it's important to find a practitioner who takes the time to listen to your concerns, answer your questions, and develop a personalized treatment plan that aligns with your health goals and values.

In addition to seeking out holistic practitioners, consider integrating other natural therapies and modalities into your Celiac Disease management plan. This may include acupuncture, herbal medicine, massage therapy, mindfulness practices, and nutritional supplements.

These complementary treatments can help support your body's healing process, reduce inflammation, and improve overall well-being. Be sure to discuss any new therapies or supplements with your healthcare team to ensure they are safe and appropriate for your individual needs.

By finding holistic practitioners and healthcare providers who support your journey with Celiac Disease, you can create a comprehensive and personalized approach to managing your condition naturally. These practitioners can help you address the root causes of your symptoms, support your body's healing process, and empower you to take an active role in your health and well-being. Remember, healing Celiac Disease holistically is a journey, and finding the right support team can make all the difference in your path to wellness.

Author Notes & Acknowledgments

First and foremost, I would like to express my deepest gratitude to the people who inspired and supported me throughout the journey of writing this book. This project would not have been possible without their unwavering belief in me and their invaluable contributions.

To my wife, thank you for your constant encouragement and understanding. Your love and support have been my anchor during the challenging times of researching and writing this book. Your belief in my ability to make a difference in people's lives has been my driving force.

I would also like to disclose that this book contains some renewed artificial intelligence-generated content. I really appreciate very recent technological innovation by outstanding scientists and of course our reader's understanding.

Lastly, I want to express my deepest gratitude to the readers of this book. I sincerely hope the strategies and methods outlined within these pages will provide you with the knowledge and tools needed to truly make your life much better. Your commitment to seeking any good solutions and willingness to explore multiple methods is commendable.

Author Bio

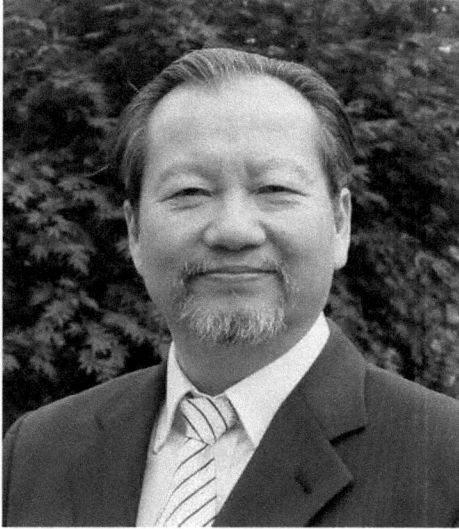

Johnson Wu earned his MD in 1982. With over 40 years of clinical experience, he has worked in hospitals in Zhejiang and Shanghai, China, as well as the Royal Marsden Hospital (part of Imperial College) in London, UK.

Upon the recommendation of Sir Aaron Klug, the president of The Royal Society and a Nobel Prize winner in Chemistry, Dr. Wu was honorably awarded a British Royal Society Fellowship. He has published medical books and articles in seven countries and currently practices medicine in Canada.

www.ingramcontent.com/pod-product-compliance
Lightning Source LLC
Chambersburg PA
CBHW060254030426
42335CB00014B/1696